THE GRANDEUR OF SLEEP™

Permission to rest.

Miraculous benefits are realized as the worlds of sleep,
relaxation and rejuvenation are explored and deeply honored.

THE GRANDEUR OF SLEEP COPYRIGHT

please note:

The written or spoken information, ideas, procedures and suggestions contained and presented in 'THE GRANDEUR OF SLEEP' workshops and books are meant for educational purposes only and is not for diagnosis. It should not be used as substitute for your physician's advice. 'THE GRANDEUR OF SLEEP' is not therapy and is not intended to replace the recommendations of a licensed health practitioner. It is the responsibility of the reader to consult with their own medical Doctor, Counselor, Therapist or other competent professional regarding any condition before adopting any of the suggestions in this book.

THE GRANDEUR OF SLEEP™

*Is dedicated to the eternal aspect
of our being which resides in the stillness
and silence of simple rest.*

MISSION STATEMENT

To guide and facilitate women
in becoming their most beautiful and radiant selves.

To acknowledge and embrace the well of love
and power which lies within all women and to ignite the
awakening and embodying of this life force.

To empower each woman, through exquisite self-care and love,
to live her fullest life possible, and to walk her path of wisdom
and truth, as she shares this light and knowledge
with all beings.

IN DEEP GRATITUDE
Thank you

The creation, birth and life of 'A Woman's Truth' would not have been possible without the love, support and devotion from the following angels in my life:

My beautiful daughter Megan who naturally embodies the teachings of living in her truth and integrity, thank you for the creative gift of the beautiful artwork. Helena Nelson-Reed for her generosity of spirit in allowing her extraordinary artwork, which embodies the teachings so magnificently, to grace the covers. Dennise Marie Keller for her unwavering support and dedication to the teachings and for proofing, editing, aligning and translating my vision into the technical world of manifestation. Dan Fowler for his creative genius and dedication. Lucy Alexander and Suzanne Ryan, my dearest friends for their amazing editing and wholehearted encouragement. Monica Marsh for her commitment, support and belief in the workshops. Maggie Crawford, my mum, for her proofing and for being a living example of the teachings. Cait Myer and Katie Steen for their patience and ability to decipher my handwriting and for formatting the books. Bethany Kelly for her support. Deborah Waring for holding the space for the conception of 'A Woman's Truth' to be born and for her insight in the first year of teaching and Emmanuel for believing in my vision.

My mentors and teachers Rod Stryker, Adyashanti and Alison Armstrong, Max Simon and Jeffrey Van Dyk for their continuous and guiding light in my life, their never-ending belief in my potential and for always teaching me the way to evolve into my highest and most potent self. And to all of you beautiful and courageous women who are committing to living your truth and transforming into your most radiant selves,

thank you.

A PRELUDE

An Overture to the Grandeur of Sleep.

What you hold in your hands is the synthesis of many years of learning, practice and teaching in the modalities of Yoga, Reiki, Nutrition, Healing and Intuition. For the years that I have known Miranda she has been a beacon of light for me in the way of healing and in uncovering that which is unseen. It is said that a true teacher leads you from the darkness into the light.

That the mastery of that teacher is in how they guide you to discover truth for yourself while equipping you with tools to dive deeper into your own healing.

Miranda is such a teacher.

The word grandeur evokes the feeling of magnificence, glory and splendor. In fact, this is what our best sleep experience should be filled with. Yet there is still so much more to be known about what exactly happens during sleep or what leads to a deep state of rest. We do know that sleep accentuates the rejuvenation of the immune, nervous and muscular systems and we certainly know what it feels like when we do not get restful night's sleep.

When we begin to craft our day to lead towards a night of peaceful sleep, we weave the quality of mindfulness into our life. The way we start our day upon waking can impact how deeply we rest that night. Starting with a meditation directly upon waking and doing some movement like yoga or tai chi is a way to create a foundation not only for your day, but also for great nights rest. What we ingest into our system in the way of nutrients, thoughts and images also plays a pivotal role in our sleep time. If we can eat mindfully, view media consciously and release negative thinking throughout the day, this is sure to pay off once our head hits the pillow.

Our deepest rest occurs during Delta and REM stages of sleep. However, those stages take at least ninety minutes to get to once we actually fall asleep. Deep sleep helps us improve our memory, reduces stress and enhances decision-making. Lack of sleep can lead to a wide range of ailments including memory problems and obesity. There are many reasons for us to commit to the practices and habits that could enhance our sleep time, besides just wanting to feel rested.

what Miranda offers in the following pages
is a beautiful guide for discovering your deepest self.

She gently encourages us to accept that we deserve to practice self-care and nurturing and lovingly offers us the tools to do so. My wish for you is that you dive into this work and discover the joys of indulging in the Grandeur of Sleep.

~ Tracee Stanley
Film Producer, Yoga Educator

THE GRANDEUR OF SLEEP™

Gems of Truth

You can download a copy of the **Sleep Declaration** and the **Sleep Study**

from Miranda's website at

www.MirandaJBarrett.com/resources/grandeur-of-sleep

A DAILY PRACTICE

commit to yourself

Follow these simple steps daily as a way to instill and strengthen your heartfelt resolve to love yourself. This will help to keep you aligned, transforming and on track, giving you a stable foundation for the rest of your life. As a gift to yourself, please mark the teachings as you read them through and congratulate yourself with each one. See each day as a commitment to take exquisite care of yourself.

You can download a copy of the **Sleep Declaration** and the **Sleep Study**
from Miranda's website at
www.MirandaJBarrett.com/resources/grandeur-of-sleep

A LIFE WORTH LIVING

"Never give from your well.
Always give from your overflow."
~ Rumi

All too often as women, your own needs are denied for the benefit of others as you orchestrate your life through demands and expectations you feel responsible for. Unfortunately, this can leave you without the juice and energy needed to be present fully and to enjoy life. During these readings, you will continually discover more about who you truly are and learn the tools needed to live your most authentic and fulfilling life possible. From this place, you will experience being 'full to overflowing' and all the joy and energy this brings.

As you delve into these teachings, you will explore, laugh, study, share, and freely express who you are. In this sacred space, you will ultimately learn your truth as a woman in order to shine, to embody your own beauty, believe in your own worth, and take exquisite care of yourself. For only in this way can you truly be of service.

During these guidebooks, many of the basic needs of women will be explored such as sleep, nutrition, creativity, movement and time to replenish. A topic has been chosen for each book and a cohesive and practical foundation is laid out to inspire and guide you. This will bring about a new strength and resolve which will allow your needs to become a priority, without letting your outer world dictate otherwise. By the end of our time together, the concept of being confident, loving, serene and passionate will no longer be a distant fantasy. Instead, these and many other extraordinary qualities that you naturally embody as a woman will flow with ease, grace and love.

With life's demands so high, it has become imperative that your needs are first acknowledged, honored and then taken care of. From this vantage point, your relationship with yourself then has the potential to be transformed into one of self-love. The beauty is this in turn creates a life that not only fulfills you and your life's purpose, but also allows everyone touched by your presence to receive this gift.

I look forward to spending this precious time with you.

Welcome to A Woman's Truth.

Sincerely and with love,

Miranda

THE GRANDEUR OF SLEEP

Sleep is ultimately a feminine pastime.

While in a sleep state, you are much more vulnerable than when you are awake. With your eyes closed and your senses shut either down or less alert, it is vital to make your sleep situation conducive to being able to relax and let go. You may have noticed when you have trouble falling or staying asleep, the harder you try, the more sleep will evade you. The beauty of the remedies in these writings is they actually create an environment that is supportive to falling asleep. Once the atmosphere is established, then sleep will naturally follow.

For a woman to succumb fully to a relaxing and deep sleep, it is vital for her to embody her feminine energy. If you are still in the more masculine mode of doing and giving, then sleep may elude you. This journey of 'A Woman's Truth' is ultimately about fully embracing the feminine power that lies deep within you, which is your birthright. It is no longer appropriate to negate or ignore this powerful source of energy or to keep pretending to be anything other than the glorious, extraordinary and powerful woman that you are. In addition, getting enough sleep is one of the most direct and potent ways to tap into this boundless supply of feminine energy.

To realize fully the amazing benefits of sleep, all you need to do is watch a baby in deep slumber. The baby reaches a profound state of relaxation. The baby simply lies there without a care in the world, relaxed, receiving life force and often with a slight smile on its lips. Compare this to the child who is overtired, screaming their head off and who cannot be appeased. This ultimately portrays the miracle of getting the proper amount of rest and sleep.

We are literally a sleep-starved nation.

In today's world, stimulation happens twenty-four hours a day; computers, televisions, shops, to name but a few. If you go back in time before the invention of electricity, the natural rhythms were dictated by the sun's rising and setting. There might have been sometime around the fireside, but at the end of the day the setting sun was a sign to rest, to go inward and to fall asleep. However, this is no longer the case.

I

Nowadays, in order for the simple act of going to bed to be accomplished, there are a number of conscious choices you actually have to make. It could be choosing not to turn on the television, the computer or the lights; but usually it is more about making the choice to turn off these devices.

How many times have you sat there in front of the television knowing you should go to bed to have the energy you need for the day ahead, but the body will not physically move? Your dedication to self-care will ultimately pull you off that couch and into bed. A part of you knows that the next hour will be many times more beneficial lying asleep, rather than slouching half-unconscious on the sofa.

The notion of 'falling' asleep actually invokes the idea of letting go, surrender, and to allow sleep to overcome you. For this state to happen, the physical, emotional, and mental bodies all need to be able to release and relax. During these teachings, you will be guided and be given tools, which will allow you to let go of each day, literally leaving it behind. Then you are ready to rest deeply and rejuvenate your whole being while you sleep. By emptying your day, you are making space for a night of deep slumber.

Have you ever noticed that when you are sick, you naturally want to lie down, rest and be still? During this time, all of your energy can go where the body needs help, whether it is fighting an infection, reducing inflammation or repairing an injury.

If you do not give your body the rest it needs,
it does not have the ability or time to heal and repair.

More and more research is being linked to the relationship between stress and illness. When you are feeling under pressure or tension, the adrenal glands are triggered and your body reacts by stimulating a 'fight or flight' mode. In this state, the body's ability to maintain the immune systems efficiency is jeopardized, because your energy is focused on the real or perceived stress trigger.

If a stress mode is maintained too long, normal physical functions that preserve a state of health are no longer able to do their job efficiently. The good news is that this can all be rebalanced by relaxation, rest and sleep, which switch off the adrenal glands and encourages the bodies systems to heal and rejuvenate.

Sleep and rest really are the most
effective and magnificent healers.

And the best part is that they are both free. No medical bills!

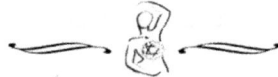

"If you saw sleep as one of the finest healers
or physician's in the world you would not
even hesitate to visit daily."
~ Anonymous

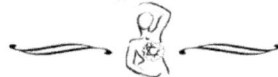

RHYTHM

A regularly recurring sequence of events.
Rhythm is a powerful natural occurrence.
It vibrates in all forms of life.
Nature flows with rhythm.

The seasons of the year evolve from one to another with wonderful regularity. Each day is followed by night, as the sun rises and sets. Even your heartbeat has its own rhythm. Without this natural occurrence, the world would be left with chaos. Disease and disorientation would prevail. It is almost as if nature or what is natural is being denied. In this dishonoring, the result is confusion and stress.

As you inquire into the definition of rhythm, it becomes clear that the sense of familiarity and expectancy that it allows is comforting. For human beings, change can often be challenging. Therefore, a regular recurring sequence of events becomes reassuring. With so much of life unknown, the rhythm of your breath, your monthly bleeding and the spring coming allows you to breathe and rest assured amidst the realms of chaos. It then makes sense to choose consciously and to follow rhythms throughout your day.

Rhythm will help support and nourish you.

Sleeping and waking are two of the most powerful of these cycles. Everyone has to sleep. It is a basic survival need. In fact, one of the most horrendous tortures is sleep deprivation because it severely goes against the body's natural instinct to rest. It is fascinating is how the world of nature supports the rhythm of sleeping and waking.

When the sun sets, the world becomes quiet and your ability to see is reduced, thus encouraging you to close your eyes. What is being suggested here is for you to follow these natural rhythms and feel the benefits they invoke and will provide you.

Jetlag is living proof of the effects of not conforming to your natural sleep rhythm; it is morning in the new time zone, yet it is all you can do, not to fall asleep over your breakfast. Another example is how out of sorts you feel the next day when you miss a night's sleep.

The gift of following nature's rhythm is that it supports and nourishes your whole system. It is the difference between planting seeds in mid winter versus the spring. It is obvious which ones will flourish and grow. As a human being, you are no different, yet when you try to overpower nature, you will end up paying a price.

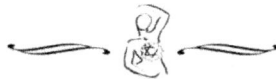

"Nature has a natural rhythm that we know and trust and because we are a part of this nature, it would only make sense to trust and have faith in our own natural rhythms."
~ Anonymous

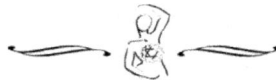

THE FOUNDATIONAL TRINITY

And in the beginning there was...

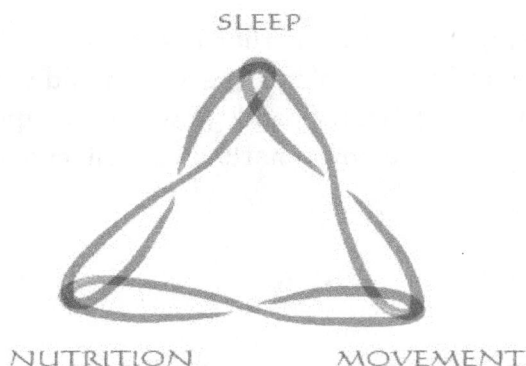

SLEEP

NUTRITION   MOVEMENT

This is the basic foundation of self-care.

By investing in your relationship with sleep, movement and nutrition, you will be infused with these essential tools which not only supply you with life force, but also give you the energy to live the life you desire. By choosing *not* to honor this 'Foundational Trinity' of rest, movement and nourishment, you place your body into a state of stress and deny the reality of what you truly need. It makes sense that a lack of sleep, unbalanced food choices or a sedentary lifestyle will not properly prepare you or your body for a day of joyful living.

Living in today's world is stressful. Yet what is being offered here is a new way of being. Instead of succumbing to the pressure of stress, listen to your bodies' voice to inform you about how you are living your life and the choices you are making.

Do not ignore stress. It is an important messenger.

Pressure and tension are sure signs that a thought experience or belief you are having feels as though it is heading in the wrong direction. Stress is your physical, mental or emotional reaction to these situations, so you must pay close attention to these feelings.

Do not shy away from them, instead lean into their guidance and message. Pause for a moment, take a breath and bring yourself back into the present moment. Allow this stillness to balance you and from this grounded and centered place be open to the possibility that there may be another choice. It may be as simple as accepting what already is, as challenging as that may be. By claiming and fully living, the teachings of 'The Foundational Trinity' your life will change. This is the groundwork needed to support the rest of your life ahead.

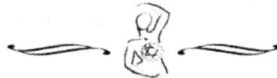

"Be careful what you water
your dreams with. Water them with worry and fear
and you will produce weeds that choke the life from your dream.
Water them with optimism and solutions and you will cultivate success.
Always be on the lookout for ways to turn a problem
into an opportunity for success.
Always be on the lookout for ways to nurture your dream."
~ Lao Tzu

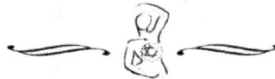

DREAMTIME AND JOURNALING

Are you women dreaming you are a butterfly
or a butterfly dreaming you are a woman?

Your dreams are your subconscious or unconscious revealing itself. With all the hubbub and commotion of daily life, much of what you are experiencing is stored with no space to be processed. This backlog can be released in your dreams.

If you pay attention to your dreams, much can be revealed. If you are dreaming that you are standing in a parched desert, dying of thirst, you could be dehydrated! By taking a moment to be still and inquire into the meaning or possible insight allows the dream to offer powerful perceptions and tools which may enhance your life. A revealing exercise is to start jotting down your dreams in a journal.

KEEPING A DREAM JOURNAL

◆ Keep a journal and a pen by your bedside.

◆ As you remember your dreams, write down the highlights.

◆ The more you do this process, the more you will remember your dreams.

◆ Ask yourself the question 'what did I dream about?' before you even open your eyes or get out of bed. As you begin to think about the day ahead, the memories can often dissipate.

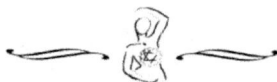

"It always amazes me how safely outrageous I can be in my dream time!"
~ Miranda

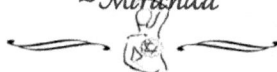

WHAT HINDERS SLEEP?

obstacles can be physical, mental, emotional or spiritual.

The following list offers some of the basic obstacles to rejuvenating sleep. Some are much easier to remedy than others are. By bringing attention to what may be in the way of a good night's sleep, you can positively affect your sleep life.

WHICH OF THESE OBSTACLES
ARE STEALING YOUR BEAUTY SLEEP?

◊ Over stimulation

◊ Overtiredness

◊ Overeating

◊ Eating just before bed

◊ Ingesting caffeine or sugar before bed

◊ Being too cold or too hot

◊ Too much light

◊ Too much noise

◊ Being uncomfortable

◊ Feeling unsafe or afraid

◊ Being disturbed

◊ Too many bodies in the bed

◊ Overactive mind or inability to relax

◊ Stress or tension

◊ Physical or emotional pain or worrying about something

◊ Falling asleep in front of the television or on the couch

9

THE EFFECTS OF SLEEP

Sleep is essential for good health and well-being.

*E*ach day you receive a certain amount of energy and when that juice is used up, a feeling of exhaustion can set in. This is especially true if you are not following the natural rhythm of your day by resting in between your 'to do' list. The good news however, is that sleep is a simple yet a highly impactful way to reclaim more energy.

◆ **Survival**

Sleep is one of the four human survival needs. If you are receiving the right amount, you will be relaxed, as your survival instinct will not be triggered.

◆ **Appetite**

When tired, the body often craves sugar, caffeine or other stimulating foods to give you energy. There is also a tendency to overeat. If you have had enough sleep, the body will not search for extra energy through food.

◆ **Vitality**

If you have not had enough sleep you will feel tired. Everything will be more of an effort or a struggle. When you are exhausted, you have a limited amount of energy to put into this experience called life.

◆ **Overall Health**

Sleep is the ultimate healer and supports the immune system and repair of the body. When you are rested, the body is less stressed and the immune system can function at its optimum.

◆ **Aging**

The more rested you are, the younger you will look and feel.

IMPORTANT FACTS ABOUT SLEEP

The body and mind need to be able to relax to fall asleep.

◆ **Sleep is one of the four basic survival needs**

Along with food, shelter and sex, sleep is what keeps the species alive.

◆ **10 pm is the Witching Hour**

Being in bed by 10 pm aligns the rhythm of the body, slowing it down to relax and rest. If you push past this time, you tend to get a second wind of energy that can keep you up for another few hours. Unfortunately, this is borrowed power and like a thief, it will rob you of the vigor you need for the following day.

◆ **The hours you sleep before midnight are worth double**

Therefore, aim to go to bed by 10 pm so you can gain the benefit of double time with the two hours before midnight.

◆ **Do not eat during the few hours before bed**

Otherwise, the body is trying to digest food rather than relax. In addition, the intakes of these calories have no way of being burned up and this may lead to weight gain. Additionally, if the food contains stimulants such as caffeine or sugar, they may well keep you awake.

◆ **Wake up naturally**

To wake up without artificial means suggests you have had enough sleep. For this to occur, you need to get to bed at a reasonable time.

◆ Relax before bed

Do not do any chores after a certain time in the evening, as this gives you at least one hour to unwind before you attempt to fall asleep. This includes working on the computer, cleaning up, doing the dishes, email correspondence, paying bills, cleaning up after children, folding laundry or whatever household chore screams for your attention.

"I make it a point to do very little after eight in the evening. I have to convince myself that the load of laundry or the email can wait until tomorrow and that giving myself some relaxing downtime with my family or myself is a much higher priority. This does not happen by default! It is a conscious nightly choice that I make."
~ Miranda

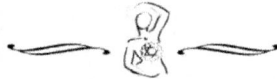

"I do not know why it should be,
but the sight of another man asleep
in bed when I am up, maddens me."
~ Jerome K. Jerome

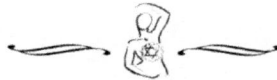

POTIONS TO HELP YOU SLEEP:

The following are some tried, tested and true remedies. Experiment with them yourself to see which ones are your own perfect medicine for a good night's sleep.

◆ A hot cup of chamomile tea.

◆ Natural Calm is a wonderfully relaxing magnesium supplement that you dissolve in hot water and drink an hour before bed.

◆ Calms Forte is a homeopathic remedy that aids relaxation and sleep.

◆ Sleep Rescue Remedy releases stress, tension and fear.

◆ Lavender Oil foot rubs relax the body.

◆ A hot bath will prepare you beautifully for sleep.

◆ Bath salts are wonderful to relax the whole body before sleep.

◆ Soaking in a pound of Epsom salts and a pound of baking soda dissolved in a hot bath relaxes the muscles.

◆ Lavender Rose cream will calm your heart and nerves.

◆ Good sex can often be a fantastic natural sleep remedy.

Remember, gratitude is the sweetest of lullabies.

YOUR SLEEP SURROUNDINGS

Allow your bedroom to become your sanctuary.

This will invite in the essence of healing and rejuvenation as you sleep, replenishing the Goddess that you naturally are.

Just as what you eat has an effect on your health and how you feel, the environment in which you sleep highly impacts the quality of your sleep.

If your surroundings have a sense of serenity and balance and nurture your well-being, this will result in a sleep life with the same qualities. Conversely, if your bedroom or sleep space is stimulating, harsh, or uncomfortable, the womb-like atmosphere needed to induce sleep will not be present.

A good example of this is the difference between trying to rest on a hard chair at the airport waiting for your delayed flight versus being in the bed you love, smothered in down quilt sand pillows, with the shades drawn, sweet silence and the hint of lavender in the air. Obviously, the difference is not rocket science!

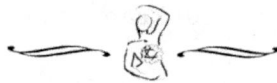

"Hope is a waking dream."
~ Aristotle

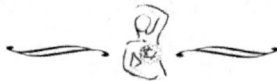

QUALITIES FOR PERFECT SLEEP:

◆ **A high quality mattress and pillow**

What you sleep on is vital. Look for a mattress and pillow that supports your back and neck and is the right firmness or softness just for you. It is important for both to be in excellent condition, relatively new, the right size and made of natural materials.

◆ **Bed linens and covers**

Choose natural materials and fibers, calming colors and textures. Make sure you have the right amount of coverings with relationship to the temperature in the room. Trying to sleep when you are too hot or too cold is always a challenge.

◆ **Sleepwear**

Sleep in natural materials such as cotton, silk, bamboo, linen or wool, as they allow the skin to breathe. Or maybe your birthday suit is your cup of tea! If you are ill, wearing a cotton or wool pair of socks can hasten your recovery and help keep you cozy and warm.

◆ **Aromas**

Using calming candles, aromatherapy, incense, creams or lotions can aid sleep. Please make sure you are choosing ingredients, which are natural and not synthetic, because what you inhale or place on your skin is ingested into your body just the same as food.

ENHANCE YOUR SLEEP ENVIRONMENT:

Feng Shui in the Bedroom.

◆ **The position of the bed**

If possible, make sure you can see the door from where you lie in bed. In an ideal world, the head of the bed would face north.

◆ **Do not place anything under the bed**

Using it as a storage unit can distort your dreamtime.

◆ **No mirrors should be placed in the room**

This is especially true at the foot of the bed. This can invite in a third party!

◆ **Limit electronics as much as possible**

Plug in or charge cell phones and computers in a different room. If there has to be a television, cover it with a natural fiber scarf or throw when it is time to sleep.

◆ **Invoke a feeling of a sanctuary**

Decorate the room in a way that provides a nurturing environment. Pay attention to the types of artwork and accessories that you bring into this space. It is important that they encourage the right atmosphere for sleep and relaxation.

◆ Sex in the bedroom

The bedroom is also a space for sensuality, sexuality and connection, so allow these essences to be present. Create an atmosphere that invites and enhances the playful, sexual and romantic side of you. Your temptress no longer deserves to live under the bed! It is time to let her out to play. With enough sleep, this is more than just a fantasy!

◆ Clutter

A bedroom is not a space to store, file or dump your belongings. Treat it as you would a sanctuary or spiritual dwelling. Keep the room clear, organized and free from objects that are not connected to sleep, relaxation or sensuality. Allow it to become a haven and space in which you look forward to entering and spending time. Imagine that!

Sweet Dreams!

A SLEEP INQUIRY

Sleep is the body's most powerful medicine.

Without enough sleep the tendency is to become impatient, and resentful of the next chore, because you do not have enough energy for the task at hand. Yet with a good night's sleep, suddenly there is a surplus of resources and the day ahead can be filled with a sense of ease, rather than resentment and anger. Becoming aware of your sleep patterns can allow you to make sleep a priority and bask in its grandeur.

ANSWER THE FOLLOWING HONESTLY:

◆ **What time do you usually go to bed?**

◆ **What do you do in the hour before bed?**

◊ Bathe or Shower

◊ Journal

◊ Pray or Meditate

◊ Contemplate your day

◊ Read

◊ Magazines   ◊ Religious or Spiritual writings
◊ Newspapers   ◊ Calm relaxing writings
◊ Nonfiction   ◊ Fiction
◊ Exhilarating or scary writings

◊ Conversation with a live human

◊ Sexual contact

◊ Stretch

◊ Feel gratitude for your day

◊ Work on and resolve any emotional issues, therefore going to bed relaxed

◊ Fall asleep while watching TV

◊ Do chores or pay bills

◊ Eat

◊ Go on the computer

◊ Vigorous exercise

◊ Go out on the town

◊ Do work-related tasks

◊ Talk on the phone

◊ Take care of children

◊ Animal care

◊ Drink

    ◊ Caffeine   ◊ Alcohol   ◊ Sugared Drinks
    ◊ Herbal tea or calming drink   ◊ Water

◊ Smoke

◊ Go to bed angry or upset

◈ What else do you do the hour before bed?

◈ Does what you do the hours before bed effect your sleep pattern?

　　◊　Yes　　　◊　No

◈ How many hours do you sleep?

◈ Do you usually fall asleep easily?

　　◊　Yes　　　◊　No

◈ What is the quality of your sleep?

　　◊　Deep and restful

　　◊　Light and easy to disturb

　　◊　Broken and restless

　　◊　Mixture

◈ Do you dream?

　　◊　Yes　　　◊　No

◈ Do you remember your dreams?

　　◊　Yes　　　◊　No

◈ Do you awake in the middle of the night?

   ◊ Yes   ◊ No

◈ What disturbs your sleep?

◈ How long are you awake for?

◈ Do you awake naturally, feeling rested?

   ◊ Yes   ◊ No

◈ Do you need to be awakened by an alarm and feel like you need more sleep?

   ◊ Yes   ◊ No

◈ How do you feel upon waking?

   ◊ Rested   ◊ Sluggish
   ◊ Replenished   ◊ Exhausted
   ◊ Alert   ◊ Irritated
   ◊ Energized   ◊ Unwell

◆ Do you nap?

◊ Yes　　◊ No

◆ How often do you nap?

◆ Do you sleep better after exercising?

◊ Yes　　◊ No

◆ What else affects your quality of sleep?

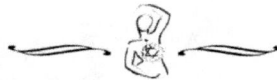

"Do not dwell in the past,
do not dream of the future,
concentrate the mind on the present moment."
~ Buddha

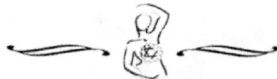

THE SLEEP EQUATION

A vital tool to receive all the energy and vitality you need.

1. **First, figure out how many hours of sleep you actually need to thrive.**

    This process will be trial and error. Try seven hours and see how you feel. Then try seven and a half or eight and see if you have more energy. You may need more sleep for a while, as you might be catching up if you have been sleep-deprived. Be patient with this process. It might take you the full month to figure out your perfect sleep quota.

2. **Second, know what time you need to wake up.**

    Even if this means you need to set an alarm clock or get someone to wake you. If you are a mother of a toddler, this part of the equation unfortunately is often dictated by their waking time, as you well know! Eventually when you are getting enough sleep, you will wake up naturally at the designated hour.

3. **Third, count backwards the hours you need of sleep from the time you need to wake up. This will give you your perfect bedtime.**

    The point is to stick to this timeline. It may differ from day to day depending on what time you have to start your morning. This means the bedtime might vary too. If you know you need to be in bed by 10 pm, which is the 'Witching Hour,' you will need to start winding down and relax at least an hour before hand; no chores, bills or emails. Spend this hour nourishing and pampering you. Maybe you will choose a hot bath or curl up with your man or second best, a good book. Perhaps a calming cup of hot tea will suit your fancy.

The equation is simple:

Time to wake up - hours of sleep needed = time to go to bed

"My daughter never ceases to amaze me when she stays up night after night until midnight doing homework and is up at six-thirty the following morning. Yet, come the weekends, if left to her own devices, which I try to allow for as much as possible, she will sleep until one or two in the afternoon to catch upon all those lost hours. The joy of being a teenager!" ~ Miranda

You know your own magic and medicine; it is all about actually giving it to yourself, making it a priority and part of your habit life.

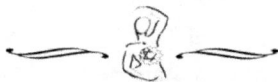

"There are times for many words and there is also a time for sleep."
~ Homer

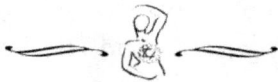

THE RICKSHAW
Releasing your day.

This is an extraordinary way to help you fall asleep and also releases much of the tension and stress of the day. As the hours of your day are reviewed backwards, it is as though you are letting go of the day's events, clearing the conscious mind.

This frees you to drop into a deep relaxing sleep and gives space for your dreamtime to reveal deeper insights, rather than coping with yesterday's experiences. The beauty of this technique is that it wipes the slate clean, then renews and prepares you for the following day.

THE PRACTICE IS SIMPLE:

◆ **While lying in bed, bring your awareness to the present moment.**

Become conscious of your position and your surroundings.

◆ **Then bring your awareness to what you were doing thirty minutes ago.**

◊ Were you brushing your teeth?
◊ Were you in the bath?
◊ Were you talking to someone?

◆ **Half hour intervals are the key.**

As you travel backwards through your day, you will get glimpses and snapshots of your life at half hour intervals. If the mind starts to wonder about the conversation at that time or the deliciousness of your lunch, gently bring your awareness back to the moment and continue to the thirty minutes before that.

◆ Keep bringing your awareness to thirty minutes before the previous time and place.

◆ Notice what you were doing and who was around you.

◆ You only need to spend a moment at each half hour interval.

◆ Reversing your day, you will bring you to that morning in bed, fast asleep.

If you are not already sleeping, chances are you will have fallen into a deep state of relaxation as the body and mind remember the previous morning's sleep state.

◆ If you fall asleep during the practice, do not worry.

The first goal is accomplished. You are sleeping!

BREATHING TO SLEEP
The Breath as a Sleeping Pill.

This yogic technique is a miraculous sleeping aid. Whenever the exhale is lengthened, it deeply relaxes the body allowing the nervous system to drop into a state of rest, therefore inviting in a sleep state. This is highly recommended on a nightly basis, as it positively affects the quality and depth of your sleep. Often, the third phase is not even reached as you have already fallen asleep.

Stage One: *Lie on your back.*

~ Inhale for a count of 4.

~ Exhale for a count of 8.

~ Repeat 4 times.

Stage Two: *Lie on your right side.*

~ Inhale for a count of 4.

~ Exhale for a count of 8.

~ Repeat 8 times.

Stage Three: *Lie on your left side.*

~ Inhale for a count of 4.

~ Exhale for a count of 8.

~ Repeat 16 times.

COUNTNG BACKWARDS TO SLEEP
Just like sheep.

If the 'Breathing to Sleep' exercise is causing stress on your system because the lengthening of the exhale feels too strenuous, this is a simpler yet just as effective technique. Again, it pulls the body back into the restful branch of the nervous system allowing the adrenal glands to switch off. A deep, restful sleep is the result.

◆ While lying in bed you are going to count backwards from twenty-one to zero.

◆ Each full breath is one count.

◆ As you inhale and exhale slowly, silently repeat the word twenty-one.

◆ On the next inhale and exhale, silently repeat the word twenty.

◆ If the mind wanders, as it will, bring it back to twenty-one and begin again.

   This is not a failure, just a sign that your mind needs more time to unwind.

◆ Keep counting backwards until you reach zero.

   You might already be asleep by this time.

REJUVENATING REST

"You are what your deep driving desire is.
As you desire, so is your will.
As your will is, so is your deed.
As your deed, so is your destiny."
~ Upanishad

Welcome to Yoga Nidra, the ancient teaching of deep relaxation. During this time, you will receive a state of calm that will replenish and rejuvenate your body. These techniques have the ability to bring you back to your center so that you will remember how to be energized. The body has an intrinsic memory and desire to be healthy. By resting and quieting the mind and the body, this desire is fulfilled.

Give yourself this gift of Yoga Nidra at least a few times a week. The beauty is the practice is done lying down; therefore, the physical body gets to be still and rest, yet part of the mind stays alert to listen to the guiding voice. Yoga Nidra can be the equivalent of many hours of sleep.

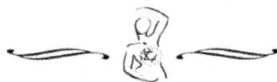

"You, yourself, as much as anybody
in the entire universe,
deserve your love and affection."
~ Buddha

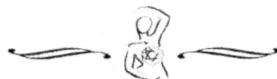

For optimum results, practice Yoga Nidra at least three times a week.

Through the guidance and teachings of the ancient discipline of Yoga Nidra, you will experience rest, relaxation, rejuvenation and a deep remembrance of the True Self. Regular use of this teaching will strengthen your resolve to live your fullest life possible. You will become the vibrant vessel you are designed to be through perfect relaxation of the physical body. By allowing the body time to lie down and deeply relax, you then allow miraculous events to unfold in your life.

It is time to give yourself the gift of these priceless teachings.

Order your copy of Miranda's CD,
'Rejuvenating Rest and the Grandeur of Sleep'.

Visit: **www.MirandaJBarrett.com**, click on the **'Shopping and Gifts'** tab and buy this unique audio journey that will provide you with the calming and restorative experience you seek.

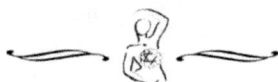

"A tranquil mind is like a single full moon shining
its brilliance on the world. Yet a disturbed mind is like the shattering
of a thousand moons as it reflects its distortion on the surface of life.
Yoga Nidra will empty your mind and allow for a thousand
moons of thought to become one."
~ Miranda

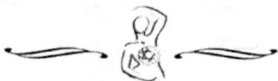

THE SIXTY ONE POINTS

Rotating consciousness throughout the body.

*T*he following is a powerful relaxation technique, which will rejuvenate your whole being. The process is simple, yet it is one of the most powerful and effective methods to reduce stress while allowing you to fall into a deep and restful sleep. As you systematically rotate consciousness throughout the body, you follow a specific method and order. The beauty is that it only takes a few minutes.

By literally following certain points around the physical body, the mind is brought to a single internal focus and each area that is thought about starts to soften and relax. Even though this practice is an ancient yogic teaching of relaxation, it could not be timelier in its benefits, as you navigate throughout modern life's rather fraught and stressful times. It seems more and more apparent how stress is a major player in the root cause of ill health. Therefore, to have an effective and potent tool to reduce this possible imbalance is a powerful ally.

"The practice of sixty one points is one of my daily practices. I often use it to quiet my mind before sleep or meditation. It is also extremely effective if I wake in the middle of the night. Literally, I will fall asleep again before I have even reached my big toe. I was given an interesting test as to its effectiveness recently. I was gifted a box of rather delicious raw chocolates which I ate way past my witching hour for caffeine. At eleven o'clock, I was stills lying there in bed wide-awake. I realized this was not going to bode well for the following day. I could literally feel adrenaline pumping through me. Therefore, with a strong resolve I began to focus my attention on rotating consciousness throughout my body. Round one seemed to switch off my adrenals. By the second round, I was asleep. Miraculous really." ~ Miranda

THE SIXTY ONE POINTS

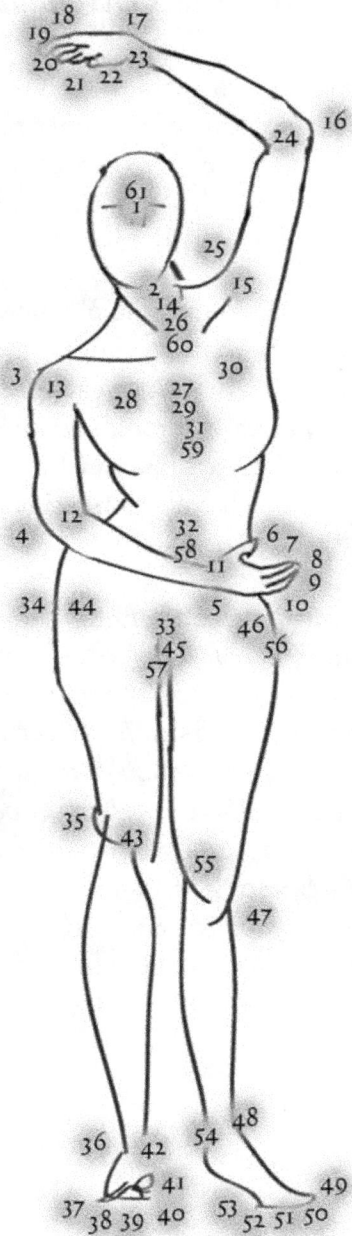

THE BOOK ENDS OF SLEEP

Begin your day as you mean to end your night and vice versa.

The hour before bed and the hour upon waking are the support system and the doorways into the quality and quantity of your sleep time and waking hours. If these two hours are honored and revered, they will greatly affect your ability to be conscious about your thoughts, actions and intentions during the following day and night. It is similar to setting a stage for the perfect, dream-come-true play that you wish to experience as your life.

THE HOUR BEFORE BED

It is vitally important to give the mind and body time to unwind before bed, therefore allowing the physical form to drop into the relaxed part of the nervous system. This will encourage sleep. How often have you tried to fall asleep when you are upset or stressed, yet to no avail? This is because the 'fight or flight' part of the nervous system is over-stimulated and is not switching off.

This precious hour is not the time to do chores, pay bills, check emails, ingest stimulating food or drink, watch something scary or adrenaline pumping on television. Also, avoid embarking on projects or conversations, which may antagonize or overly excite you. Again, this can greatly hinder your ability to get a good night's rest.

Instead, choose calming and nourishing activities such as a hot bath, a calming cup of tea or a good book. This will permit the mind and body to prepare for sleep.

THE HOUR UPON WAKING

◆ **Keep the first hour of each day as calm and peaceful as possible.**

Do not overfill or overachieve in this time. Treat it along the same vein as the hour before bed. For those of you with children, this can be challenging! If possible, awaken a little before them in order to ground and align yourself for your day, even if it is only for ten minutes.

◆ **Once you are getting enough rest you will begin to wake up naturally.**

This is a sign of your sleep life coming into balance.

◆ **Spend a few moments feeling a sense of gratitude for your life.**

This could be as simple as being thankful for the new day or being specific, such as giving thanks for your health, your relationships or your family and friends.

◆ **Roll over onto your right hand side to get up.**

This aligns the body for taking action for the day ahead.

◆ **When you get out of bed, place both feet on the floor at once.**

This helps to ground you.

◆ **Go to the bathroom.**

Take plenty of time to eliminate the toxins from the day before and you sleep.

◆ **Drink at least one glass of room temperature water on waking.**

This will rehydrate the body. Hot water and fresh lemon juice is another possibility. This will help the body to detoxify. Do not drink water that is left by your bed all night. Water is a natural conductor and can pick up negative energies that were being processed in your dreamtime. You do not want to re-ingest them.

◆ **Set your intention for the day.**

Allow your energies to align with how you desire to live out your day, before life takes on a mind of its own.

◆ **Spend some time each morning in:**

◊ Prayer

◊ Meditation

◊ Spiritual writings

◊ Journaling

◊ Movement such as Yoga or Thai Chi

◊ Stretching or dancing

◊ A walking meditation

◆ **Any of these practices can be done before bed.**

By living out these choices, you will enhance, align and replenish your essential Self and this will give you the vitality to navigate you through the day ahead.

RESTING WHILE AWAKE

permission to nap.

Just as the bookends of sleep and the importance of the hours before and after you wake up have been explored, it is also vital to pause, rest and nurture yourself during the hours between sleep.

How often have you ploughed through your day, literally existing on fumes to complete your *'to do'* list and the demands of what life is throwing at you? Unfortunately, it seems as though the permission slip that allows a woman to rest throughout her day may be missing from the female psyche.

Therefore, the first step is for **you** to give yourself permission to rest. This may be easier said than done. If a part of your self-worth and self-esteem is connected to accomplishing your tasks or taking care of people, then some down time will not only seem counter-productive but also self-indulgent or selfish.

The 'Wonder Woman with a *'to do list'* will resist the idea that replenishing yourself can actually provide you the juice you need to accomplish the tasks on hand. This permission to rest could be as simple as curling up in a chair to read a book for twenty minutes, sitting out in the sun, taking long luxurious naps or practicing Yoga Nidra in the middle of the afternoon. Whatever the choice, the point is that you stop running, pause long enough to become still and rest the physical miracle called the body. This amazing instrument is then allowed to regroup, replenish and gather the energy needed to complete the day.

"Sometimes I work in the evening. If I orchestrate my day well and lovingly, this will mean that I have some quiet down time in the afternoon or a later start in the morning, so I am not demanding a twelve-hour, nonstop day of myself. What I notice is that if I have the space to lie down on my bed and practice Yoga Nidra for thirty minutes, I rise as a new woman. I then have energy for the evening and instead of willing myself through the work, I am energized and passionate again. On the other hand, if I do not have the space to pause and rest, I still turn up, but the life force is no longer in me and my sense is that neither I, nor my clients truly benefit." ~ Miranda

REVEAL MORE TRUTH

Without sleep, you are but a mere shadow of your true self.

As you utilize these tools and teachings remember that your ultimate goal is to create an exquisitely sacred space for yourself the hour before you go to bed and the hour upon wakening. Invoke the feeling you might have upon entering a place of worship. One rarely brings one's *'to do'* list to church unless your intention is to surrender it to a higher power. If that is the case, go for it! If not, keep those thoughts out of this space and treat yourself with sweetness and kindness during this time of rest and rejuvenation.

By following and living out these suggestions, your sleep will be enhanced and enriched, which in turn will highly benefit you in your waking hours. For those of you who would just like to pop a pill and fall asleep here is the next best thing.

THE FOLLOWING ARE SIMPLE INVITATIONS
FOR YOUR COMMITMENT OF LOVING YOURSELF:

◆ Read your entire book more than once.

It makes good bedtime reading!

◆ Set a daily intention upon waking.

Bring in the quality of gratitude and keep the intention simple and direct. This will bring you clarity as to how you want the character of your day to evolve.

Examples are:

◊ May my day be filled with Blessings, ease and grace.
◊ May my actions be filled with love, light and higher guidance.
◊ I accomplish my Divine Mission and Purpose throughout this day.
◊ I am given what I can handle and I am able to handle what I am given.
◊ I choose to take exquisite and beautiful care of myself.
◊ I am deeply grateful for my life.

◈ **Please be mindful to maintain and strengthen your loving and inspiring intention.**

Remember this is a moment in time to cultivate and strengthen your Truth.

◈ **Throughout this exploration of sleep, be loving, kind, and generous to yourself.**

This is a learning process. Most importantly, you must forgive your mistakes.

◈ **Go to my website at www.AWomansTruth.com to print out copies of your sleep chart so you have at least four-week's worth.**

Keep the chart by your bed with a pen. Religiously fill it out each morning. Let go of your hang-ups about school and teachers and getting your homework in on time. This is ultimately a gift to yourself and will reveal huge insights into your sleep patterns and habits, the good and the exhausting!

In life, it is always important to discern
if your daily choices give to you more than they take.

◆ **Use the sleep equation to figure out how much sleep you need each night.**

Your sleep chart will help you with this.

◆ **Each night practice a different method, which aids falling asleep.**

Counting backwards, Breathing to sleep, 61 points, Rickshaw or Yoga Nidra. Practice in this case may not necessarily bring perfection, yet it will invoke a more loving, patient and vital you.

◆ **Fill in your Sleep Declaration.**

Once you have a sense of your own personal sleep patterns and rhythms, you can declare your commitment to maintaining this healing process. **Go to my website at www.AWomansTruth.com to print out copies of your Sleep Declaration.**

There is a saying that suggests:

we become an expert when we have explored,
failed and succeeded many times over in a very focused field.

At this point, it would probably be safe to say that everyone is an expert on sleep. 'A Woman's Truth' is about turning the tide and starting to put some new expertise into practice. As you attain a new level of consciousness around your own personal sleep patterns, you can become your own sleep Guru, which in turn will invoke and empower the Feminine within you.

Allow forgiveness to be a conscious part of every one of your days. Remember, at any given moment you are doing the best you can. Let go of what was, release what cannot be, and accept what is. Have compassion for yourself.

The rhythm or routine that you establish for yourself is worth its weight in gold. Just as you have noticed with young children, they feel safe and secure when they have a set rhythm and routine before bed. Your life force will also react to the practices that you choose to set for yourself. Sometimes the mere act of washing your face and brushing your teeth, subtly, but powerfully, sets the space for sleep. Be mindful of these rhythms and know that by adhering to them, your task will be more easily accomplished.

This 'Truth Work' comes to you through deep reverence for the work, dedication, and consciousness that you are embarking upon. You are changing the tide for womankind and blazing a new trail. Remember you have a lifetime to change and cultivate your relationship with sleep. It will be a daily step-by-step process that will make the difference. Be kind and loving with yourself.

This will ultimately help you fall asleep! I look forward to connecting with you in the next chapter of your life as we explore **'Nourishing Nutrition'** and reclaim your health and vitality.

I wish you the sweetest of dreams,

Miranda

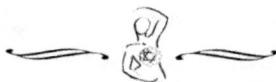

"A well-spent day brings happy sleep."
~ Leonardo da Vinci

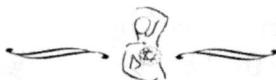

CHARTS, CHARTS, GLORIOUS CHARTS

"A good laugh and a long sleep
are the best cures in the doctor's book."
~ Irish Proverb

This Sleep Chart will bring a new level of awareness and consciousness to the foundation of your life. It will give you clarity on what is working and what is not.

◆ Please go to **www.MirandaJBarrett.com/resources/grandeur-of-sleep** to print out more copies for yourself. Give yourself the gift of seeing your life clearly laid out in front of you.

◆ Fill out the **Sleep Study** on a daily basis until you begin to see your patterns and how much sleep you truly need.

◆ Ask yourself the powerful question: Is your sleep life giving you more energy than your life is taking away?

◆ Once you are clear about your basic sleep needs and see the importance of honoring this vital aspect of your life, make the necessary adjustments to lovingly replenish and nurture yourself.

◆ Once you have discovered how to be rested and energized, you are now ready to fill in your **Sleep Declaration**. This is a commitment of love and tenderness.

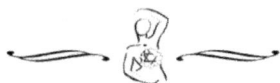

"Finish each day before you begin the next,
and interpose a solid wall of sleep between the two."
~ Ralph Waldo Emerson

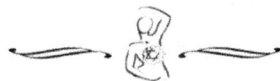

SLEEP STUDY

Give yourself the gift of seeing
your sleep life clearly laid out in front of you.

DAY	Did you nap or rest in the day?	How long before bed did you stop your daily routine?	Did you eat close to bed time? If so what?	What did you do the hour before bed? *	What time did you go to bed?	How many hours did you sleep?	How did you feel upon waking? *	What was the quality of your sleep? *	What else may have affected your sleep time?
MONDAY									
TUESDAY									
WEDNESDAY									
THURSDAY									
FRIDAY									
SATURDAY									
SUNDAY									

For words and descriptions, see the Sleep Inquiry chapter, page 18, in this book.

Please go to
www.MirandaJBarrett.com/resources/grandeur-of-sleep
to print out more copies for yourself.

A LIVING DECLARATION OF SLEEP

And a daily commitment to self- care.

I, _____

declare that

I need _____ hours of sleep a night to flourish.

I choose to be in bed by _____pm
to be present fully and vital for the following day and to wake up naturally.

I will stop doing chores and work by _____pm
therefore having time to unwind, relax, and prepare for a deep, restful sleep.

In the hours before bed, I choose to:

_____

_____

Thus I feel nurtured, nourished, ready and prepared for sleep.

I decide to do at least one of the following each day
so I am fully able to embody my feminine power:

Meditate, nap, Yoga Nidra, sleep practices,
go to bed early, unwind or spend time alone.

I choose to do this out of a deep love and tenderness for myself.

Signed with love,

_____

ABOUT MIRANDA

A spirited guide and mentor.

Miranda is a passionate and devoted leader. Her loving and wise support will guide you on a transformational journey as her powerful teachings unveil the truth of who you are. Her gift is to offer potent tools, which inspire exquisite and beautiful self-care and empower you to live the fullest and most authentic life possible. As a mentor and guide, Miranda deeply walks her talk and is fearless about her own path of self-discovery, as she weaves the sacred into the mundane.

The simple, yet powerful premise offered by the mystic Rumi is the foundation of Miranda's philosophy and mission:

> *"Never give from the depths of your well,*
> *always give from your overflow."*

Miranda gives Council and Guidance for the Mind, Body and Spirit. With a background in Nutrition and Energy work, Miranda is the Creator of 'A Woman's Truth' and 'The Spirit of Energy', an Author, a Workshop and Retreat Leader, a Reiki Master and Yoga and Meditation teacher. Miranda studies under the guidance of her Beloved teachers Rod Stryker and Adyashanti.

To speak with or follow Miranda, please call or visit:

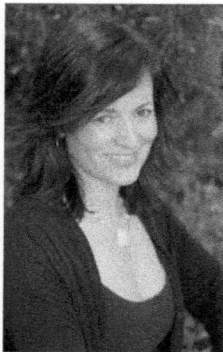

Phone: 626~798~6544
eMail: Info@MirandaJBarrett.com
Website: www.MirandaJBarrett.com
Facebook: Miranda J Barrett
Twitter: MirandaJBarrett

ABOUT HELENA

A visionary artist.

Helena Nelson-Reed is a visionary artist whose primary medium is watercolor. Born in Seattle, Washington, she was raised in Marin County and Napa Valley, California and today lives in Illinois. A largely self-taught artist whose educational emphasis and degree is in psychology, Nelson-Reed's primary focus is exploring the collective consciousness and the portrayal of archetypal imagery in the tradition of Carl Jung and Joseph Campbell. Rendered in luminous watercolor technique often described as ephemeral, Nelson-Reed's paintings are created in extraordinary detail, pushing the medium of watercolor past the usual limits. Her work may be found in private collections, book covers, magazines and CD covers. Nelson-Reed also has a line of jewelry, calendars and greeting cards.

Helena's Mission:

My images can be interpreted many ways, and for some will serve as portal to the mythic landscape. Descriptions providing background about each painting are available by request. Navigating and translating myth into contemporary wisdom is the traditional way of transmitting information, a shamanic and multi - cultural practice.

Myth, fairy, folk and spiritual lore describe divine beings and supernatural life forms arriving unbidden and disguised. In our earthly dimension, mortals often play similar roles in the lives of one another. Destinies and energies collide and interact, visible and invisible forces are at work. The mythic realms are timeless, offering insight and inspiration. While my paintings have a positive energy, many have roots in the shadows of life experience and human psyche; like the lotus blossom rooted in pond mud. For many, life is one challenge followed by the next, like beads on an endless string.

Take heart! Like goddess Inanna, one may navigate the underworld, move through dark places yet return to the realms of light battle scarred but wiser, richer for the experience. Read the ancient tales, the great mythic literature; draw strength, for they are repositories of wisdom.

Visit Helena's website for her art purchase information and art to wear jewelry:

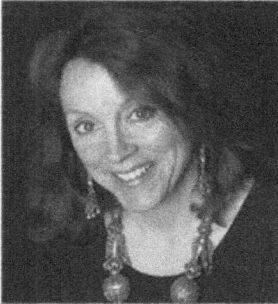

eMail: HNelsonReed@Gmail.com
Websites: www.HelenaNelsonReed.com
www.etsy.com/shop/HelenaNelsonReed
Blog: www.dancingdovestudio.blogspot.com
Facebook: MorningDove Design By Helena

MIRANDA'S WORLD

*ways to stay connected
and aligned with your truth.*

BOOKS:

A Woman's Truth

A life truly worth living.

Priceless teachings reveal your transformational
journey ahead. Obstacles to self-care are explored
as clear and loving intentions are conceived.

The Grandeur of Sleep

permission to rest.

Miraculous benefits are realized as the worlds of sleep,
relaxation and rejuvenation are explored and deeply honored.

Nourishing Nutrition

Reclaim your health and vitality.

Reap the bountiful rewards while eating as nature intended.
Claim your health and vitality with these simple,
yet powerful tools to nourish and heal your body.

Embodying Movement
Ground your whole being.

Restore balance in your life. Discover how to embrace
your whole being through the life-enhancing benefits of body movement.

Body Care
Cherish your body as a temple.

Learn to honor your extraordinary body
as a living temple and listen to the healing messages she whispers.

Feminine Power
Fully access your supreme birthright.

Welcome and reclaim this intrinsic privilege while living
in harmonious balance between the masculine and the feminine.

The Abundance of Wealth
Receive the gifts of prosperity.

Understand the energy flow of prosperity and weave
the threads of abundance throughout the tapestry of your life.

Find Your Authentic Voice
The courage to express who you truly are.

Your greatest ally is born
when you courageously speak your truth and claim your unique power.

Loving Yourself
A love affair with the self.

As you become highly attuned to your own needs,
allow love to lead the way. Grant yourself permission
to honor and express your heart's truest desires.
Love yourself, no matter what.

Living A Spiritual Life
Ground your divine essence here on earth.

Discover what spirituality means to you, by consciously
living between the two worlds of the sacred and the mundane.

Service As A Way of Life
Ignite the fire of love to truly be of service.

By utilizing the gems of exquisite self-care
on a daily basis and honoring your truth, your mission of service is born.

The Crowning Glory
Fully Rejoice in Being You.

A celebration overflowing with love,
blessings, grace and gratitude. Stand confident within
your truth as your mind begins to serve your heart.

The Food Of Life
The versatile vegetable.

More than just a cookbook,
a comprehensive guide for nourishing your life.

Reiki
The spirit of Energy.

An insightful guidebook full of wisdom
which introduces you to the potent and healing world of Reiki.

CARDS:

Inspiration Cards
A daily Spiritual Practice.

Sixty-Five cards with simple yet inspirational qualities
to live by and an insightful guidebook to lead the way.

CD'S:

The Grandeur of sleep
and Rejuvenating Rest

An ancient healing art of rest and relaxation.

Simple yet profound practices that alleviate stress and tension
allowing your mind, body and spirit to heal, restore and replenish.

TO ORDER PLEASE VISIT:

www. MirandaJBarrett.com
www.Amazon.com

All books are available in printed or eBook form.

TESTIMONIES

to 'A Woman's Truth' teachings.

"As an educator and a life-long learner, I am drawn to the anecdotes and metaphors of life. So when I am curious about a word such as its origin, its usage, its syllabication, its definition, I turn to a dictionary; but when I am curious about myself, the origins of my beliefs, identifying the best usage of my talents, the 'chunks' that make up me, the definitions of who I am, I turn to Miranda and 'A Woman's Truth'. It is there, within the loving comforts of her conscious care, where I can take risks, share unabashedly, listen compassionately, challenge thoughtfully, and grow intuitively. 'A Woman's Truth' sets you on personal journey to learn how to love and embrace the many different layers of the feminine."

Kelsey ~ Teacher ~ Altadena, CA

"I am so very grateful to Miranda for reconnecting me with my power. 'A Woman's Truth' is for courageous women ready to face their issues. I had to unlearn much of my conditioning to find and make room for my truth of loving myself."

Monica ~ Artist and Mother ~ South Pasadena, CA

"These guidebooks gave me the time and a safe place to look at all aspects of myself and my life. At age 71 I realized it was not too late to change and grow, so I could continue helping others by taking care of myself first. After completing these twelve 'A Woman's Truth' books, I am excited and very grateful for the gift that Miranda has given me through the teachings."

Maggie ~ Director of Non Profit ~ Pasadena, CA

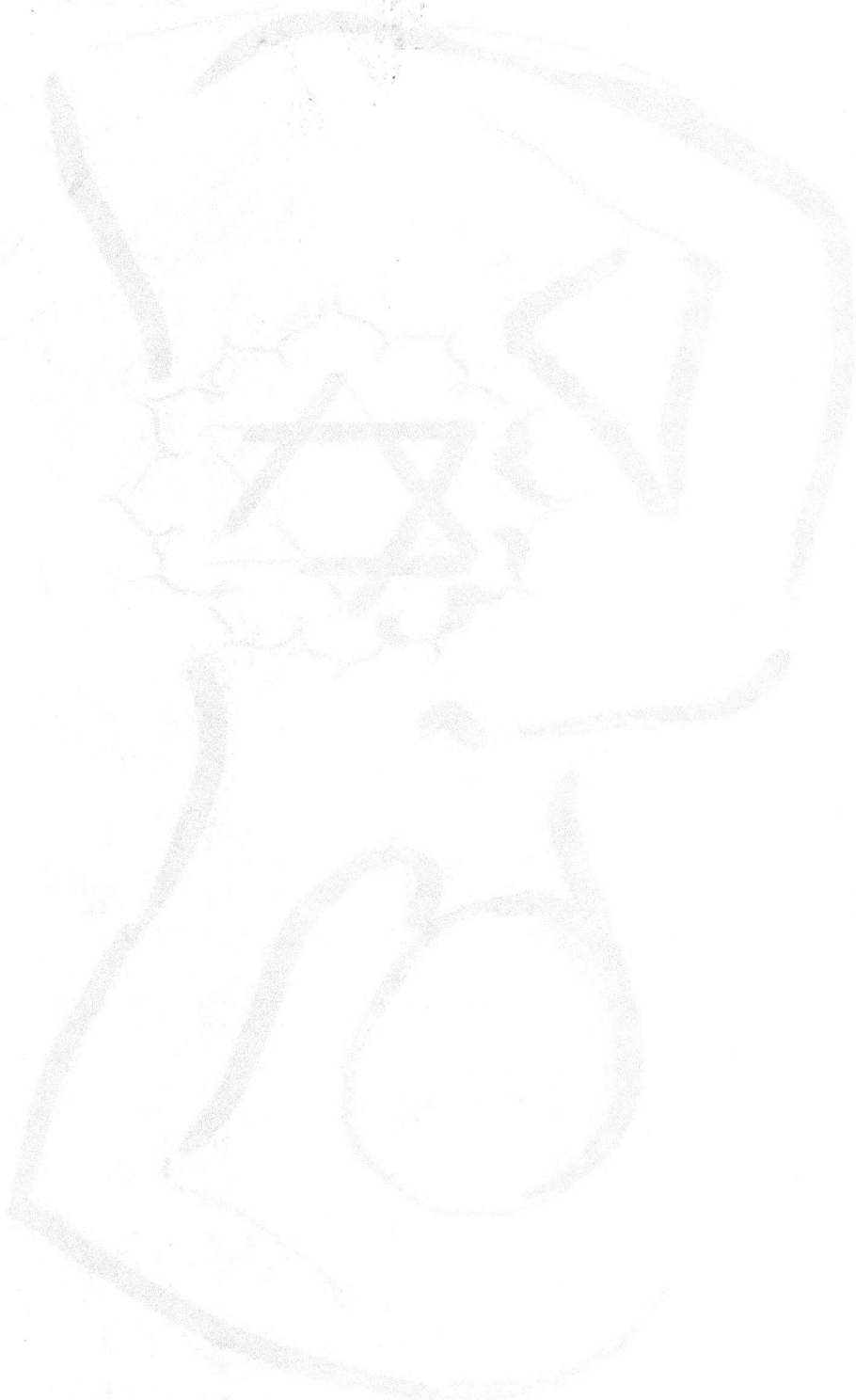